Using Coffee Enemas to Improve Health

Ryder Management Inc.

Prologue

"Let food be thy medicine and medicine be thy food."
Hippocrates

"You only live once, but if you do it right, once is enough."
Mae West

.

Table of Contents

Prologue   iii

Table of Contents   v

Introduction   1

The Gerson Therapy   3

Coffee Enemas and Detoxification   5

About Coffee Enemas   7

What is Glutathione   9

Benefits of Coffee Enemas   10

Performing the Coffee Enema   12

Enema Tips and Techniques   15

Closing Remarks   19

About the Author   21

Introduction

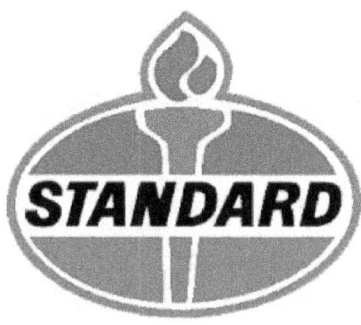

Did you know that one 42 gallon barrel of oil only creates 19.4 gallons of gasoline? The other half of that barrel of oil is used to make over 6,000 other common household items including, but not limited to: clothing, cosmetics, deodorant, petroleum jelly, detergents, insecticides, hair die, perfumes, candles, antihistamines, food preservatives, shampoo, toothpaste, aspirin, plastics, pharmaceuticals and just about every other household product used on a daily basis. In fact, petroleum products are so entrenched in our life; we don't even realize how deep it goes. Since the beginning of Rockefeller's Standard Oil Cartel, by incorporating petro-chemical or petroleum by-products into the manufacture of a company's product, companies were assured the kick back grants and subsidies offered. Since these toxic chemicals are in everything we consume, is it any wonder the functioning of our liver becomes impaired?

Chemicals have permeated every aspect of our lives to the point where the average person has hundreds, if not thousands, of different carcinogenic, industrial, domestic and agricultural chemicals built up in our bodies.

Never has this planet been as polluted as it is today. The laws of most nations permit the addition of over 3,000 chemicals in our food, health and healthcare products.

Coffee enemas have the ability of removing these toxins from our bodies.

.

The Gerson Therapy

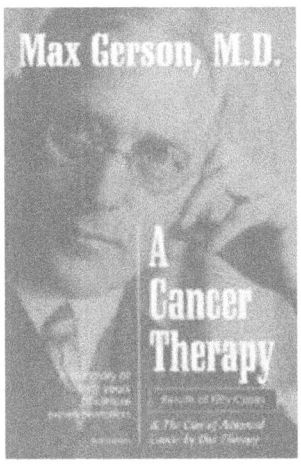

Born in Wagrowiec, Germany on October 18, 1881, Dr. Max Gerson was an American physician who developed "The Gerson Therapy", an alternative method for treating cancer and other degenerative and chronic diseases. *The Gerson Therapy* is based on the belief that disease is caused by the accumulation, in our bodies, of a number of poisonous substances and toxins.

The Gerson Therapy is a natural treatment that activates the body's extraordinary ability to heal itself **by incorporating a plant based diet, raw juices, natural supplements and coffee enemas.** This powerful natural therapy boosts the body's immune system and has been used to successfully heal terminal patients with cancer and other degenerative diseases.

After Dr. Gerson's death on March 8, 1959, his youngest daughter, Charlotte, continued to promote the Gerson Therapy, founding the Gerson Institute in 1977. Do see their website at Gerson.org.

Coffee Enemas and Detoxification

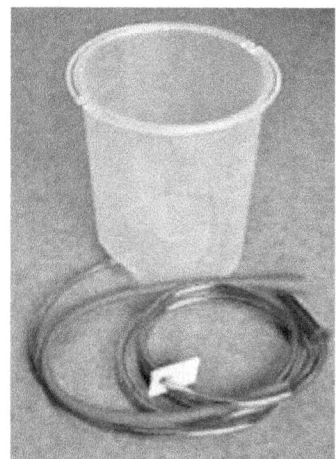

Enema bucket with catheter
Gerson.org

During World War I in Germany, shortages were experienced with respect to medical supplies and pain medication needed to treat casualties of the war. In order to help soldiers manage their pain after surgery had been performed, nurses discovered that administering coffee enemas into patient's rectums greatly helped to relieve pain, in the absence of pain medication such as morphine.

After the war ended, two German scientists studied the effects of administering coffee into the rectum of lab animals. They discovered that the caffeine would enter the liver through the hepatic portal system and cause an increase in the flow of bile. The bile, in turn, would accumulate the poisons and toxins in the liver and subsequently release them from the body upon evacuation.

Did you know that Mae West (August 17, 1893 – November 22, 1980) was a great believer in the benefits of daily coffee enemas and started every day with a morning enema? Many people say that this ritual is what contributed to Ms. West's vibrant and bright personality and glowing attractiveness.

About Coffee Enemas

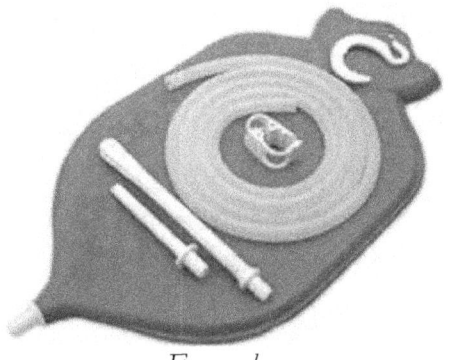

Enema bag

The purpose of coffee enemas are not that of improving elimination, rather, their purpose is to stimulate the liver into releasing, and thus removing, accumulated toxins in the liver along with removing free radicals (which cause cell damage) from the bloodstream.

Coffee enemas also have a specific effect on the colon which has been observed through an endoscope. Coffee enemas cause dilation of the bile ducts, causing a greater production of bile which in turn makes it easier for the liver to breakdown and excrete toxins.

Coffee contains *palmitic acid* which has the effect of stimulating the production of *glutathione S-transferase* (GST) and other ligands. This enzyme group reacts with free radicals in the bloodstream making them inert. These neutralized substances are then dissolved in the bile, then released through the bile flow from the liver and gallbladder and ultimately excreted through the intestinal tract. Glutathione production is regarded as an important mechanism for carcinogenic detoxification.

According to Dr. Gerson, introducing 32 fluid ounces of a coffee solution into the colon will first dilate portal blood and then bile ducts. Two other major constituents of coffee, namely theophylline and theobromine, counters gut inflammation in addition to dilating blood vessels.

Blood in the body passes through the liver every three minutes and by retaining the coffee enema for a period of at least 12 -15 minutes, the coffee enema becomes a form of dialysis of the blood across the gut wall.

.

What is Glutathione

Glutathione is an antioxidant enzyme and is often referred to as the body's "master antioxidant" since it is primarily responsible for protecting the body's cells from free radical damage. Glutathione is made up of the amino acids *cysteine, glutamine and glycine* and is mainly found in the liver, but carries out its function throughout the body.

The level of glutathione in the liver is critically linked to the livers ability to detoxify. When we are constantly exposed to toxins such as chemicals found in everyday products, toxins in cigarettes, chemicals in pharmaceuticals and pesticides on our food, glutathione in the liver is significantly reduced, thus impairing the liver's ability to function properly.

Glutathione deficiency contributes to oxidative stress, which in turn plays a key role in aging and the onset of diseases such as liver disease, Alzheimer's disease, cystic fibrosis, cancer, heart attacks, diabetes, and more.

Studies show that increased glutathione production greatly improves liver function.

Coffee enemas increase the production of glutathione by as much as 700% in the small intestines which facilitates detoxification of the liver. Palmitates (chemicals in coffee) and caffeine work synergistically to stimulate and cleanse the liver and blood.

Benefits of Coffee Enemas

Those coping with a chronic degenerative disease or an acute illness can expect to obtain the following benefits after administering coffee enemas on a regular basis:

700% reduction in toxicity;

Improved blood circulation;

Improved immunity and tissue repair;

Enhanced tissue health;

Increased cell energy production;

Cellular regeneration;

Reduced pain and pain management;

Nausea relief;

Relief of general nervous tension;

Reduced depression and bad moods;

Increased energy levels and improved mental clarity;

Improved digestion;

Increased good gut bacteria and reduced bloating;

Elimination of parasites and candida;

A cleansed colon by removing fecal impaction;

Helps to rebuild the liver;

Increased pH or alkalinity of the entire intestinal tract;

Improved hydration;

Improved skin health;

Relief of constipation;

Improved sleep;

A reduction or softening of frown lines;

Yang effect;

Coffee enemas are one of the best detoxification methods for health and beauty.

Indications of an Impaired Liver:

Increased digestive issues such as food cravings;

Constipation, gas, indigestion;

Bad breath or bad tastes in your mouth;

Headaches and migraines;

Feeling older including epic hangovers;

More aches and pains;

Angry outbursts for no particular reason;

More noticeable frown lines and bad moods;

Serious health issues such as diabetes or other autoimmune disease;

Weight gain, especially around your middle;

Acne, dry skin, rashes

If you are experiencing any of the above, you should consider administering a coffee enema.

Performing the Coffee Enema

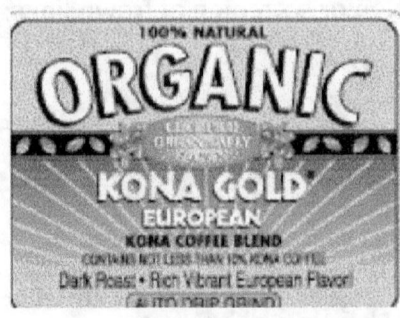

Drinking a cup of coffee has an entirely different effect on our bodies relative to that of using caffeine in a cleansing enema. In addition to efficiently eliminating the buildup of toxins in the liver, coffee enemas also provide a quick relief from fatigued and malaise.

Prior to preparing your coffee enema, it is recommended that you read this book in its entirety.

The following provides a starter list of the essential supplies necessary for performing a coffee enema at home:

Purified or distilled water, just over one quart (four cups)

Ground organic coffee is highly recommended and should be stored in your freezer to maintain maximum freshness.

BPA free 48 ounce enema bucket with catheter tubing (available at Gerson.org) or a similar sized enema bag

Lubricant such as coconut oil for lubricating the tubing and rectal area;

Towels, pillows, music, watch/clock and/or book/magazine/tablet to enhance comfort.

To prepare the coffee enema: put a little over one quart (four cups) of clean distilled water into a sauce pan and bring to a boil.

Slowly stir in two tablespoons of ground organic coffee, and continue to boil uncovered for five minutes. This will drive off the oils. Cover with a tight fitting lid and continue to simmer for another 15 minutes. Turn the heat off, leaving the pan on the burner; allow it to cool to body temperature before using.

Using a coffee filter, cheese cloth or other straining device to strain the mixture into your enema bag or bucket adding additional distilled water to bring the quantity up to 32 fluid ounces. Your enema is now ready to administer.

Determine where to perform your enema, such as the bathroom floor or even in the tub. Once you have decided where, prepare the area in a way that is comfortable and relaxing for you by setting out towels, cushions, pillows and/or padding.

Lubricate about two inches of the plastic tube (that will be inserted into your rectum) with coconut oil along with lightly lubricating the entry to your rectum and surrounding area with coconut oil. Coconut oil has the added benefit of being anti-bacterial and anti-viral.

Prior to inserting the tube into your rectum, let the solution run through the tube and into the sink or toilet to remove the air and any air bubbles.

With the enema bucket placed at least 18 inches above you, such as on the bathroom sink, while lying down on the floor, insert the tube about two or three inches into your rectum and then turn to lie on your right side. Open the clamp and allow the fluid to run slowly into you while you relax and breathe deeply. If you can, retain the fluid for at least twelve to fifteen minutes before eliminating on the toilet. Retaining the fluid for the full 12-15 minutes may be difficult at first. Don't worry about this as most people have to administer a number of enemas over the course of a number of days, in order to obtain this.

Once you expel the enema, you will probably need to eliminate again, usually after another twenty minutes from expelling the coffee.

If you are unable to release the enema as a result of a congested abdomen or dehydration, a second enema may be taken immediately after the first one. However, DO NOT do more than two consecutive enemas in a four hour period. At least four hours must be allowed between double enemas.

It is important that your equipment is thoroughly washed and cleaned after every use by using a mild detergent. This must be done after every use as the bucket and tube would otherwise become an excellent growing environment for bacteria and other germs.

After washing your equipment thoroughly, spraying with a 6% diluted solution of food grade hydrogen peroxide (FGHP) is a natural and effective way to ensure your equipment remains clean and germ free.

Quick Brew Method

If time is short, you may benefit by the "quick brew method" of preparing your coffee enema as follows: place 2 tablespoons of organic coffee in a coffee filter, held in a strainer, placed over a cup. Add hot distilled water. Add this cup of coffee to your enema container. Add three more cups of purified water. This will reduce the temperature to a comfortable level to use immediately.

Enema Tips and Techniques

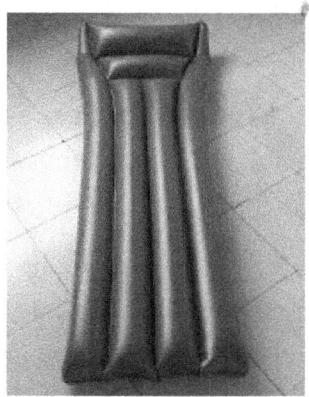

The easiest place to perform the enema is in the bathroom. Determine the best place for you to lie down and then cover the area with blankets, towels or a mat.

You will want to prepare your area to enhance your comfort and relaxation. Items for this purpose may include a cushion or pillow, reading material, a glass of water, a scented candle and comfortable clothing such as a robe.

Have a clock or watch nearby in order to time the 15 minutes.

Use coconut oil to lubricate both yourself and the tubing as it is antimicrobial.

While holding the enema in your rectum, massage your abdomen in a counter clockwise direction to help the solution move higher into your colon.

Lie on your right side for five to ten minutes before turning to your left side for an additional five to ten minutes.

If you initially have difficulty holding the enema, take the enema in two batches. This should make it easier to hold the second enema longer when just beginning with this practise.

If cramping is an initial problem, experiment with dilution: both quantity and temperature. In other words, you may find that adding more coffee, more water or adjusting the temperature can make the enema more effective for your body.

A medium or dark roast organic coffee has been found to restore blood levels and glutathione more effectively than light roast coffee.

If intestinal gas is a problem, bending and stretching exercises before the enema may help. Alternatively, an initial enema of only distilled water or chamomile tea, before your coffee enema, may also help reduce or eliminate gas.

A bowel movement before your enema will help you hold the enema longer.

Drinking plenty of water and fresh juice before and after your enema to replenish hydration is important.

It is normal to hear or feel a squirting out and emptying of the gallbladder. This occurs under the right rib cage, or sometimes closer to mid line. If after a week of daily enemas you don't experience this, you should consider making the coffee stronger by increasing the tablespoons used by ½ a tablespoon per quart of water, but not exceeding two tablespoons per cup. Alternatively, you may only need to increase the amount of water used.

For optimal health, your goal should be the ability to retain the quart or divided into two enemas of half a quart each (two cups) for up to 12-15 minutes each. Never force yourself to retain it, if you can't.

After performing the coffee enema a few times, you will get better at holding the enema for the minimum time of 12-15 minutes.

This time period (the 15 minutes retaining the fluid) is perfect for meditation, reflecting on positive thoughts and even working through and removing built up negative emotions.

This time period is also a good time to do natural vision exercises for improving natural eye sight.

The Gerson Therapy recommends up to five coffee enemas per day for chronic diseases such as cancer.

Performing an enema once a day or a few times each week is ideal for maintaining health and beauty.

Ensure to periodically run boiling water, hydrogen peroxide or other comparable antimicrobial agent, through the empty bag or bucket and tubing to discourage mold growth when the equipment is not in use.

Closing Remarks

Ancient healers have recommended coffee enemas for thousands of years. A description of enemas can be found in the Dead Sea scrolls, which date back at least 2,000 years. The coffee bean and plant have also been a part of herbal medicine and healing for hundreds of years in the west.

Between the years 1899-1977, coffee enemas were included in the Merck Manual, only being removed to make room for new material. The Merck Manual has long been considered the Bible for Physicians.

Today, liver detoxification is more important than ever before. As a result of chemicals and toxins contained in our food, cosmetics, soaps, shampoos and even the air we breathe, we are being poisoned on every conceivable front. In addition, all the prescription and over the counter drugs we consume also have serious consequences on our health. With this in mind, it is no surprise to learn that our liver can become overloaded with toxins, sludge and stones, impairing its ability at removing these poisons on its own. If toxins get backed up in our liver and are then unable to move through the digestive system to be excreted, they will be reabsorbed back into the body and stored in every imaginable place making disease and chronic health inevitable.

The Gerson Therapy is a non-specific treatment that effectively treats many different conditions by healing the body as a whole, rather than selectively targeting a specific condition or symptom. Over the past 60 years, thousands of people have used the Gerson Therapy to recover from so-called "incurable" diseases, including: Cancer, Diabetes, Heart Disease, Arthritis, Auto-immune disorders, and so much more". The Gerson Therapy incorporates coffee enemas, a vegan diet, raw juice and vitamin supplements to reverse chronic and degenerative disease.

I sincerely hope that this book has provided value to you. If you enjoyed this book, please tell others, if not, please tell us.

info@RyderManagement.ca

About the Author

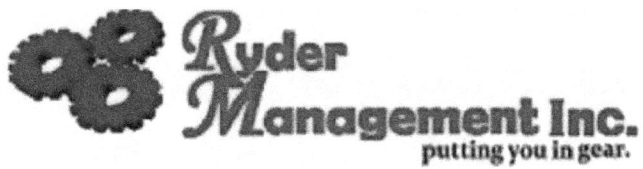

Ryder Management Inc. (Rydermgt or RMI) is a Canadian Controlled Private Corporation (CCPC) based in London, ON Canada. As an "umbrella" organization, RMI brings together a group of authors whom are professionals in their respective fields and are writing with the primary goal of providing books that educate, comfort and offer assurance that natural health remedies do exist and are an effective and safe way to regain, obtain and maintain our health.

Please see Ryder Management Inc's author page at Amazon: http://www.amazon.com/Ryder-Management-Inc/e/B00ICGMCRS

for other books written by Ryder Management Inc.